Yourfitnesssuccess.com

Resistance band Training

A Resistance Bands Book

For Exercise At Home

Or On The Go.

James Atkinson

CONTENTS

Section 1

Why resistance bands?

Resistance bands are an amazing piece of home gym equipment, and everyone who shows the slightest bit of interest in fitness and exercise should own some form of resistance band training equipment.

Resistance band training is so versatile and can fit into everyone's training routine regardless of fitness goals and differing levels of ability. Resistance band training can be used by:

> Total beginners to fitness and weight loss
> People who are in rehab after injury
> People who are working on mobility and function
> People who just want to get their body moving
> People who want a tough circuit training session
> Endurance trainers
> Bodybuilders

The scope for resistance band training is as broad as the fitness and exercise industry itself.

Now we know that resistance band training is for everyone, we can talk about the versatility of this type of exercise. One of the major draws to exercise band training is that if you own a standard set of exercise bands and a modicum of knowledge on how to use them, you technically have a personal gym with everything you need to complete a substantial, full-body workout that fits conveniently into a small bag. You can store your "full gym" in a draw or cupboard and you can easily take it with you if you want to train on a business trip, on holiday, at work on your lunch break at work... Or there is a pandemic on and all the gyms close!

These things are absolutely fantastic and I can't say enough about them! I will, however, finish by saying that they are very inexpensive for what they are and you can pick up a quality set that will last you years for around the price of a single month's gym membership or a single session with a personal trainer!

So you have heard my opinion on resistance band training and probably established that I am a firm advocate, but who am I and what gives me the right to set about creating a guide on the subject?

My name is James Atkinson (Jim to my readers and friends). I've been into fitness and exercise for most of my life and my experience has an extreme range, from skinny to competing bodybuilder, from fat to endurance runner, I have formal qualifications in advanced fitness instruction, am an Amazon bestselling author in the fitness niche.

This information is not an excuse for me to brag, but I believe it's essential for you to know some background on the author of potential exercise advice that you intend to follow. At this point, I want to thank you for your purchase and let you know I am always willing to help where I can with your fitness journey.

I'd also like you to know that I am a real person, (not a ghost writer) I'm passionate about my subject and write from personal experience, I have had great success with fitness but part of the journey to great success is often great failure and I have that too and I share a lot of this too.

If you do struggle with anything fitness or exercise related, please shoot me over an email at admin@yourfitnesssuccess.com I'll do my best to help where I can.

The bottom line is that I want you to get results and I'm here to help you get to where you want to be in fitness!

Follow Along In Real Time...

In the second half of this guide, we will go through several different exercise set ups along with a section on how to create your very own personalised routine. Knowing how to change up your exercise programme to suit your goals is a valuable skill and this will become easier with more experience of training. If you would like to get serious right away, fully commit and get to where you want to be with fitness and weight loss as soon as you can, I have you covered!

I have created a six week, progressive video course that's based on home workouts and resistance band training. The main aim of the course is to offer a solution to the beginner that covers everything from planning, prep, goal setting, motivation and mind-set all the way to actually following along with me in real time on screen and training for results in your own home.

Results in fitness and weight loss have always been my driving force. This goes for me and for my personal training clients. I want everyone to hit their fitness and weight loss goals, so I've designed the home workout for beginners video course to do exactly that!

We will work on a weekly basis, the first week is really an important week where we lay the foundations, we'll sit down and start planning for success, well find our motivation, get specific about our goals, I always advise making these goals ambitious because we can all achieve more than we think we can!

Week 1 through to week 6 is where we hit our home workouts! Each week is more progressive than the last. We build on our training from the previous week by tweaking the exercise choices, adding intensity and further challenging ourselves. Some people develop quicker and can move from week to week seamlessly, but the beauty of this course is that if you find a week a bit too challenging, you can repeat the previous week. Everyone moves a different pace so it's no problem!

So if this sounds like something you are interested in, please check out the video testimonials, check out the sample videos and you can even start the course for free!

It would be great to see you over at:

YourFitnessSuccess.com

Home   About   Blog   Podcast   Frequently Asked Questions   Contact   Member Login

Online Home Workout Courses

Fitness results
you can count on!

No gimmicks, no fads, just real advice with results in mind.

Let's do this!

START THE COURSE FOR FREE

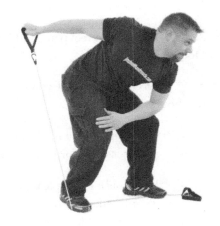

What do others think about this course?

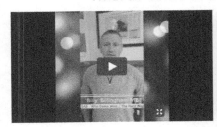

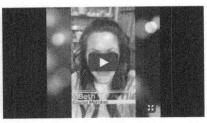

"Far more than your usual fitness video training! This is a serious, progressive exercise course!"

Health Check

Before you embark on any fitness routine, please consult your Doctor or physiotherapist. If you have any health conditions, always check if the type of exercise and exercise choices you intend to involve yourself with.

1.   Do not exercise if you are unwell.

2.   Stop if you feel pain, and if the pain does not subside, consult your Doctor.

3.   Do not exercise if you have taken alcohol or had a large meal in the last few hours.

4.   If you are taking medication, please check with your Doctor to make sure it is okay for you to exercise.

5.   If in doubt at all, please check with your Doctor first – you may even want to take this routine and go through it with them. It may be helpful to ask for a blood pressure, cholesterol and weight check. You can then have these taken again in a few months to see the benefit.

Which resistance bands?

There are lots of types of exercise bands out there. Some are designed for specific body parts and exercises; some are made of fabric, some of latex, some of elastic. Some are tubular, some are flat, and the list goes on. There are also many resistance bands that are essentially the same product but are marketed to a certain group, so this is something to be aware of.

When you look past all the noise and marketing, there are only really three types of resistance band. The loop band, the stretching band, and the resistance band made for attachments.

The loop band

The loop band is normally a flat circular band made of either latex or fabric. These can often be found in sets of varying tensions and sizes or can be bought as a single unit. This type of band is usually recommended as an aid for stretching, rehab or other more specific training, but they can be used for all other types of training if you have the right tension band along with the knowledge of how to utilise it.

As these are essentially a loop and they are designed for specific exercise choices, you will find these in many sizes. An example of this is that you may see a loop band designed specifically to aid in pullups. This will be a fairly large loop. You may also see one designed with outer leg exercise in mind. These will be a much smaller loop than the one designed as an aid to pullups.

The stretching band

These bands are normally made of latex or elastic and are available in many lengths. The key feature that sets these apart from the other two is that they are flat and tend to be much wider. These bands are normally used as an aid in the development of flexibility and function, often the physiotherapist's choice for rehab. The wide surface area is very useful for better purchase when performing raised leg exercises and using bare feet as an anchor point.

As these are flat, you will tend see and hear them referred to as a "roll", and as they are often used for rehabilitation, you may also hear them called "rehab bands".

The exercise band set with attachments

These are widely available and are probably the most versatile. They are usually tubular bands of varying tensions that have small hooks at each end. These hooks are used to transform the band into a specific piece of exercise equipment. As well as the exercise bands, these kits normally contain several handy attachments, such as stirrups for hand placement, a door anchor and ankle cuffs for lower body exercises.

Each exercise band can also easily be turned into a loop band by linking the two hook ends together, and they can also be stacked onto the attachments if you outgrow the highest tension band in your set.

Which one do I recommend? There is no reason you can't own variations of these bands. The more you have access to, the more scope you have for exercise. If you only wanted to invest in one type of exercise band, however, I would recommend that this was the "exercise band set with attachments". This has the most versatility, as you can create loop bands, add attachments that turn the band into a piece of exercise equipment for a specific muscle group, you can stack them and these exercise band sets usually include a compact bag for storage and transportation.

If you are using resistance bands for home workouts, these kits also usually come with a "door anchor". This means that you can perform some fantastic exercises that target specific muscle groups so you can directly work on your weak parts or problem areas. If you have access to one of these kits, you have all the tools to mimic the resistance movements of many of the exercise machines in your local gym. There is a lot of scope for full body exercises too.

I have no affiliation to any company that make these exercise band sets so I will not point you in a direction but they are easy to find and widely available across a broad price range, so have a look around and pick one that suites you to get started.

This is an example of one of these sets with the attachments:

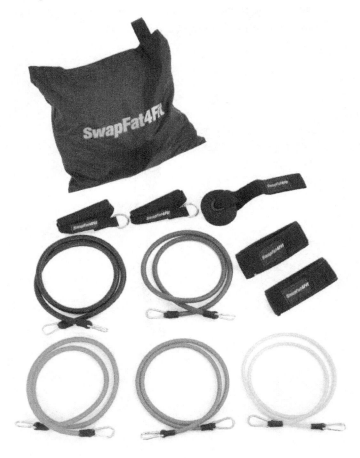

When using a set like this in conjunction with this book, it is entirely possible to simply utilise the bands without any attachments, and when performing some exercises, this is preferable. But having the handle attachments or "stirrups", connected can be more comfortable and can mimic holding dumbbells.

More advanced trainers can also use these stirrups to attach multiple bands to increase the resistance if the thickest band in the set doesn't present enough of a challenge for progress when performing certain exercises.

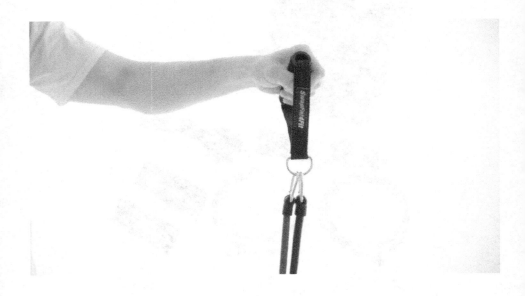

The door anchor is used for many exercises in this guide and is a really useful piece of kit. It can be placed at the top of a door to create tension from above for pull down type movements or at the bottom to create tension for pull up type movements. Ankle straps also feature. These can be strapped around the ankles and used in conjunction with door anchors for leg exercises. You should expect to see one door anchor, two ankle straps, and two stirrups in a good kit. Here is a picture for reference:

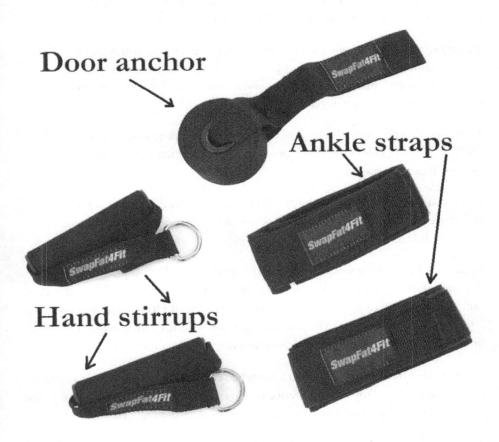

Door anchor

Ankle straps

Hand stirrups

An important lesson in exercise

Whether the exercise method you are doing is cardio based, resistance based, is of a rehabilitation nature or a mixture of everything, you should always make sure you are getting the most out of it.

To get the most out of any exercise, you must understand what the movement or exercise method is designed to do and make it count when performing it.

The more you know about any subject, the better equipped you are to excel at it, and the same goes for exercise and fitness. If you understand why you are performing a certain exercise, you execute it with good form and stay consistent with your training, you will get results.

Many people join a gym, buy a fitness book, or hire a personal trainer to get fit and lose weight. This is the first step, and it's a hugely important one, but this alone will not get results.

Once you are in the gym, you have a fitness guide or in this case you have a resistance band workout plan, you need to take a bit more into consideration if you want results.

In the late 1970s there was a documentary created called "Pumping Iron". This documentary is not only responsible for the fitness industry as we know it today, but it was also the catalyst to much creation in terms of Hollywood movies in the 1980s, and so much more. The documentary was also my introduction to weight lifting, and it is what sparked my interest in the industry too.

I've seen this film enough times to know the script from memory, as in my early training days; it was my only reference on how to train with weights. There is one scene in this documentary that I remember to be my first real takeaway.

The scene starts with a close-up of a motivated gym member questioning whether he needs more weight on a barbell that most people could not lift off the floor. The star of this shot soon decides it's a definite yes, and he hurries out of the camera shot.

The camera is then conveniently left pointing at the ample midriff of a seemingly very unmotivated late twenties/ early thirty something male going through the motions of a set of single arm dumbbell bicep curls using, at a guess 2.5 kg dumbbells. This does not look like it's challenging him, he is out of shape; he is obviously in the gym because he wants to change, which is great, but the inclusion of this shot by the filmmakers is most definitely to prove a point.

After lingering on this shot for a while, the camera then switches to our original star. He has loaded his extra weight onto the bar and is ready to start his set of barbell shoulder press. The bar is on the floor, loaded with what I estimate to be close to, if not 100kg.

He sets himself up by bending over the bar and taking a shoulder width grip, you can hear, see and even feel his determination as he psyches himself up before cleaning this bar to his chest with good form and proceeding to smash out ten reps of shoulder press.

He reaches exhaustion and says out loud with a grimace,

"No more!"

Then something takes over, and he manages two more reps before dropping the bar onto the floor and saying,

"I'm not satisfied! I want more weight!"

We as the viewers are left feeling exhausted! We have also learned an important lesson; if you want to look like the original hulk, you have to train like him! If you are in the gym and you are cruising, you may as well not have signed up.

Firstly, I want to address the fact this is an extreme example, but the more extreme the example, the more stark the point of the anecdote.

The next disclaimer is to point out that this is not to bash the guy in the gym who's out of shape; I have a lot of respect for anyone who takes the steps to join a gym or start a fitness routine. It can be an extremely daunting place!

It's no surprise that as a young, uneducated fitness beginner, this scene was one of the most influential to me. Even though it is a short, seemingly bland scene compared to the rest of the movie, it showed me that if you want to get results;

you need to put the effort in! You need to be motivated and you need to work hard! If we set aside the fact that this focuses on a champion bodybuilder in a bodybuilding world, the principals stand for every form of fitness training.

By going to the gym myself, I would later learn that it's not just pushing yourself, lifting heavy weights and training to exhaustion every session that counts, but there are more important things you need to prioritise. Training hard and challenging yourself is a must if you want to earn any type of result, but exercise form is something that should be the number one concern to any trainer.

Once you choose a method of training and the exercise choices for your training program, you should learn the movements. Make sure you understand what this exercise is supposed to be doing for you. What muscle groups the exercise targets, what function of the body you are working on, how you should breathe during the exercise and, while you work on this, be aware of how challenging the movement is for you.

A competing bodybuilder once told me that once you step into the gym, you should have left your ego at the door. This is a statement that I didn't appreciate until I'd been training for a while. He was talking about lifting heavy weights. Sure, lift heavy weights to get stronger and to progress, but be lifting those weights with correct form. If it's too heavy for you and you are just counting reps without thinking about form, you are not getting the most out of your training session, not to mention, you will open yourself up to injury!

The last thing I would like to address here is that I am also aware that training with resistance bands is not just for getting lean, toned, strong and fit, but some trainers will use these movements for rehabilitation after injury and for function, movement and maintenance. So whether you are looking for aesthetic changes, improved muscular and joint function or general wellbeing from a resistance band workout, always make sure that your exercise form for each movement is as good as it should be.

So if you want to get results and make your workouts count, challenge yourself, but do so with perfect exercise form.

Exercise methods. Which is right for you?

There are lots of ways that you can train for lots of different outcomes. One of the best things about resistance training is that you can take the same handful of exercise choices and use them to get these different results.

You can take squats, chest press and shoulder press and use these exercises to build muscle mass and strength, and you can use the same exercises to train for endurance or fat loss. The difference is in the method of training that you choose to do.

Although resistance band workouts can be used for many situations, they are an excellent choice for fat burning and muscle toning exercise goals.

For fat loss and muscle toning, there are several effective methods of training and, depending who you are and what your experience with exercise is, there are varying approaches.

There is a progression with training methods for fat loss and body toning. If you are a total beginner to exercise, the progression with training methods will be as follows:

Single exercise (sets and reps)

In this method of training, we would focus on a single exercise for several sets with rest between each set before moving on to another exercise choice and doing the same.

Example – Resistance band chest press 3 sets of 12 reps before moving onto resistance band squats for 3 sets of 12 reps and so on until we have worked through all the planned exercise choices for the workout.

Timed

Training for a set amount of time is another common method of exercise. This is often done by performing exercise sets within a time range. For example, squats are performed continuously for 30 seconds, there is a short rest period, and then another 30 second set of squats is performed. This can be used for every exercise in a routine or it can be used for specific exercises only.

Supersets

In this method of training, we would select our exercises for our training session, but instead of focusing on a single exercise, we would perform two. One immediately after the other.

Example – Resistance band chest press for 12 reps and then immediately onto 12 reps of resistance band squats, then we would have a short rest. This is known as a "superset". We would then repeat the superset several times before moving onto another superset using two different exercises.

Circuit training

In this training method, we would perform one set of every exercise choice that we have selected for our training session, with no rest between exercises. Once we have finished the last rep of the last set, we will have completed one circuit. This can be repeated several times.

Circuit training is a fairly intense method of training and is also a short, sharp way to get effective fat burning and muscle toning exercise sessions done.

As you can see, circuit training and superset training may not be a good idea for the beginner as these sessions can become pretty intense, dependent on the exercise choices and volume but there is always an easier progression to be used as a stepping stone to these methods of training.

If you are a beginner, start with the single exercise method of training and run this for several weeks before moving onto supersets for several weeks and finally on to circuit training. Of course, if you have a preference to any of these methods of training, you can stick to that one and just challenge yourself with other variables like changing the resistance level, rep range, etc.

If you are not new to exercise, have no health issues or injuries, you can jump right into superset training, circuit training or a combination of all three, but please remember exercise form is important, and it's always better to be cautious with volume and intensity of exercise when you are starting out. If it's new to you, take it easy at first to gauge your body's reaction to the training.

Your exercises, your way

In the second section of this book, there are Twenty-one different exercise choices listed with illustrations and descriptions. There are three choices for each major muscle group and also a few bonus, all over body exercises for more advanced and intensive training.

Exercise is a personal thing and although there are plenty of "one size fits all" exercise routines that are very effective and will work for most people, there are also instances where many people will find some exercise choices and methods of one of these programs difficult to adjust to or perform altogether.

Although I have created several "one size fits all" programs based on the exercises and methods outlined in this guide, I have also created a system of sorts In this book so you can create an exercise program that suites you by either tweaking one of my "done for you" routines or creating your own from scratch.

If you are going to follow one of the routines that I have already created, great! But if you would like to create your own, here are the steps to follow:

Decide on the training method

The first step is to decide on the training method. Revisit the chapter on exercise methods and have a look again at the methods of training mentioned there. Are you ready for a circuit training session? Do you want to start with a single exercise focus for sets and reps or do you fancy training in a superset style? Maybe you want to train three times per week and try a different method in each session. If this is the case, create three programs, one for each training method that suites your needs and ability.

Choose your exercises

Exercise choice is the next consideration. Once you have decided on your training method, you now need to add in some exercises. If you are going for full body workouts, I would suggest that you select at least one compound movement for each body part. Try to also include at least five exercises per session. You could also choose to focus only on certain muscle groups per session by choosing several exercises per body part. Have a look at the exercises choices in the book, read the descriptions, become familiar with the target muscle group and select the ones that you want to add to your workouts.

Choose your intensity and workload

You have your training method and exercises, now you need to decide on the intensity and workload. The more reps that you do in a set and the more sets that you do, the higher the intensity and the more resistance you add, the bigger the workload.

A good starting point is 3 – 4 sets of 10 – 15 reps per exercise with a resistance band that becomes challenging at 8 reps onwards. This is a standard, entry level approach to the "single exercise focus" method, but there is no reason you can't add more sets and reps or use less. With superset training and circuit training, you can also use this rep range.

When choosing the resistance level, aim for an exercise band that challenges you enough for you to be working the muscle throughout the set, but it's not so heavy that you can't perform the exercise with good form.

Write it down.

Once you have got all of this in place, make it official by writing it down on your own program card. If you've not done this type of thing before, you'll soon see how useful it is to have your own exercise program written down in front of you while working out.

Exercise program cards

Once you've decided how you'd like to train, you can put your exercise plan together!

I've created a blank program card for each training method for you to copy, fill out, and jump right in. There are also complete examples of each training method for you to take inspiration from, switch out some info to suit you better or use as they are.

It's always a good idea to know why you are doing what you are doing, so if you would like to know what the thought process was behind the creation of each of these routines; this is also there for you to take ideas from and is well worth the read if you are interested in creating effective routines for yourself.

I have created these example routines with myself in mind. Because of my background, qualifications, I know my strengths and weaknesses; this gives me an advantage when designing routines, but the thought process behind creating these workouts should shine light on some factors that you may not have considered.

Everyone's different and you have to start somewhere, but the longer you train for, the wider the variety of training methods you try, the better you will connect with your own body in terms of exercise, strengths, weaknesses and your ultimate goals. You will also be better equipped to create effective exercise routines for yourself.

SINGLE EXERCISE

MUSCLE GROUP	EXERCISE	RESISTANCE BAND	SETS	REPS
Chest	Chest press	Red	3	12
Back	Lat pulldown	Blue	3	12
Legs	Squats	Black	3	12
Front of arms	Bicep curls	Blue	3	12
Back of arms	OH Tricep extension	Red	3	12
Shoulders	Shoulder press	Blue	3	12
Abdominals	SB Crunches	Body weight	3	20
------	------	------	------	------

Why this routine?

This is an all over body routine that targets one muscle group per exercise. This would be a great workout for a beginner or someone who wanted to maintain or hit a quick home workout between gym sessions or as a substitute for the odd missed gym session.

Muscle groups

The order in which to train the muscle groups is not an accident. With full body routines like this one, I would always follow an order similar to this one. The idea is that you start with a small muscle group, have the big ones in the middle and then back to a smaller group, but always finish with abs and lower back exercises if you choose to include these.

Exercise choice

As this is an all over body workout, I have included mostly "compound exercises". These exercises are big movements that hit more than one muscle group per rep. Examples of compound movements are Chest press, squats and shoulder press, any exercise that requires multiple joints to perform correctly.

Resistance band

The resistance bands that I have are colour coded to match a resistance level. In the resistance band set that I have, I normally only need to use three. Red has the least resistance, then blue is a fair bit tougher and black has the most resistance. I am familiar with the intensity of these bands and what challenges me adequately on each exercise, so it was easy for me to fill in. If you are unsure about your resistance levels, you will probably need to test these out for a few sessions before finding your flow.

Sets

I have chosen to go with three sets as I would train with this routine three times per week. If I were planning to use this routine exclusively over several weeks, I would look to increasing this to four sets. But three sets is a good starting point.

Reps

The rep range is set to 12, as this gives me a decent amount of time working each muscle. If I decide to up the resistance of the exercise bands, I can aim for failure at the tenths rep and maybe use "cheat reps" for the last two. "Cheat reps" is a term used in advanced training and bodybuilding and this fits my goals, but 10 – 12 reps is a good rep range to aim for with all over body workouts. The last note on this is that I have chosen 20 reps with abdominal exercises. This is because abs can be trained to "reasonable failure" and my reasonable failure with these exercises is around 20 reps.

"Reasonable failure" means continuing to perform reps until you can't complete another rep in good form.

CIRCUIT TRAINING			
MUSCLE GROUP	EXERCISE	RESISTANCE BAND	REPS
Chest	Chest press	Red	12
Back	Lat pulldown	Blue	12
Legs	Squats	Black	12
Front of arms	Bicep curls	Blue	12
Back of arms	OH Tricep extension	Red	12
Shoulders	Shoulder press	Blue	12
Abdominals	SB Crunches	Body weight	20
-------	-------	-------	-------

NUMBERS OF CIRCUITS	-	3
REST BETWEEN CIRCUITS	-	2 minutes

24

Why this routine?

This type of full-body workout is designed to effectively develop muscle tone and promote fat loss and is an excellent choice for anyone looking for a short, sharp workout with that goal in mind. This can also be used as a substitute for other types of workouts to mix things up a bit, or it can be used exclusively.

Muscle groups

The muscle groups, exercise choices, resistance bands, sets and reps have been chosen to reflect the "single exercise" training method. This is not only to show how easy it is to turn your "single exercise" routine into a circuit in order to progress to circuit training, but to also show you a way to take the exercises that you are familiar with and turn your routine into a short sharp fat burning circuit.

Exercise choice

Although I have shown a circuit training session using familiar exercises for a full-body workout, it is possible to do many things with circuit training. For a start, you could add more exercises to make the circuit longer or use several exercises choices for the same body part to give more focus to that area.

Resistance band

It's possible to complete a circuit using the same resistance bands as you would in other training methods, but a point to note here is that the extended, continuous nature of this training means you will probably fatigue a lot quicker finding it harder to use a workload that you would use with other training methods.

Sets

"One set" is known as "one circuit" in the world of circuit training, but each set contains several exercises.

Reps

When choosing the rep range of each exercise, it's important to keep in mind the amount of exercises that you are adding to your circuit. More exercises means more reps. A good starting range in terms of reps and sets ratio is 3 sets of 8 – 12 reps. This, however, will depend on the individual and the fitness goal.

Rest between circuits

Depending on the size of the circuit and rep range, a circuit can put a lot more demand on the trainer, so you will need varying amounts of rest between circuits. I would recommend at least one minute rest between sets, but no more than three. Too much rest can cause a trainer to cool down or fall out of the desired training heart rate zone, making the session less effective.

SUPERSETS				
SUPERSET	EXERCISES	RESISTANCE BAND	REPS	SETS
#1	Chest press	Red	12	3
	OH Tricep extension	Blue	12	
#2	Squats	Black	12	3
	Seated calf raises	Black	15	
#3	Shoulder press	Blue	12	3
	Lateral raises	Red	12	
#4	Bent over row	Black	12	3
	Bicep curls	Blue	12	
#5	Lower ab crunch	Body weight	15	3
	SB Crunches	Body weight	15	
#6	Squat & row	Blue	15	3
	Squat & shoulder press	Blue	15	
#7	------	------	------	------
	------	------	------	

Why this routine?

This type of training method can be used as part of a single exercise routine to target certain muscle groups with more intensity. It can be used for full body workouts, split training or blitz training so it's pretty versatile. In this example, I've chosen a full body routine.

Muscle groups

In this example, I've chosen to either superset two exercises that complement each other from a functional view (an example of this is "Chest press & OH tricep extensions"; the triceps are also worked in the chest press movement) or chosen two exercises that hit the same muscle group (Shoulder press & Lateral raises).

Exercise choice

Where there are supersets of compound movements and isolation movements, I always have the compound movement before the isolation. This is because the compound movement uses more muscle groups. It's a bigger movement and my goal is to stay strong. This means I am fresh for a strong set with a higher strength resistance band. If my goal was to become more toned, I would put the isolation exercise first.

In this superset routine, I've also chosen to add two big, double movements at the end of the workout. This will make the session a lot more intense. It's unnecessary to do this as these muscle groups have already been worked, but this is a great way to add value to your workout if you are a more advanced trainer.

Sets

Each set is effectively 24 reps, but my goals are to stay strong and build up so I will work with the resistance band that I would use in a single exercise method. This will add intensity to the workout. 3 sets will also be the target for each superset. This can be moved up to 4 for extra progression. I will also reiterate here that this routine is an advanced example. The training volume is high and some exercise choices are for more advanced trainers.

More training plans to play with

Here are some more ideas for exercise routines. Again, these can be used for inspiration, tweaked to fit your personal fitness goals better or followed directly. The exercises have been added to the following routines, but the sets, reps and resistance band s have been left out as this depends on your training goals. The exception to this is the first exercise routine that shows a timed training method. These figures are simply used as an example and can be changed accordingly.

FULL BODY TIMED ROUTINE

MUSCLE GROUP	EXERCISE	RESISTANCE BAND	SETS	SECONDS
Chest	Chest press		3	20
Back	Lat pulldown		3	20
Legs	Squats		3	20
Lower Legs	Seated calf raises		3	20
Front of arms	Bicep curls		3	20
Front of arms	Drag curls		3	20
Back of arms	Tricep extension		3	20
Shoulders	Shoulder press		3	20
Shoulders	Front raises		3	20
Abdominals	Elevated Crunch		3	20

UPPER BODY ROUTINE				
MUSCLE GROUP	EXERCISE	RESISTANCE BAND	SETS	REPS
Chest	Flys			
Chest	Chest press			
Back	Lat pull down			
Back	Row			
Front of arms	Bicep curls			
Front of arms	Drag curls			
Back of arms	Tricep extension			
Back of arms	Tricep kickbacks			
Shoulders	Lateral raises			
Shoulders	Shoulder press			

MUSCLE GROUP	EXERCISE	RESISTANCE BAND	SETS	REPS
quads	Squats			
Glutes	Kick backs			
Outer leg	Leg abduction			
Legs/back	Deadlift			
Lower leg	Calf raises			
Lower abs	Lower ab crunch			
Abdominals	Exercise ball crunch			

Section 2

Introduction to section 2

Here you will find a whole range of exercise choices with multiple options for each major body part. There are at least two illustrations of each exercise that show the starting position and end position of each movement. These illustrations also show correct posture. Posture and the way you hold yourself during exercise is extremely important, so please have this at the forefront of your mind when practicing and performing all exercises.

Along with the illustration of each exercise, there is a description. If you are new to exercising or even new to exercising with bands, take the time to read through the exercise descriptions and familiarise yourself with the movement. It's best to have a go at the exercises and make sure you can perform them correctly before getting into the actual workouts.

There are three exercise choices for each major body part; Chest, Back, Legs, Arms and Shoulders. Two bonus categories are also present at the end. The first of these is a few choices for the Abdominal muscles if you would like to add these into your workout and some double movements that make for great progression options or to add something more challenging into your workout.

If you are up for creating your own exercise routine, go ahead and copy the blank exercise tables if you are reading the eBook version, or if you are reading the paperback, just fill them in!

SINGLE EXERCISE				
MUSCLE GROUP	EXERCISE	RESISTANCE BAND	SETS	REPS

CIRCUIT TRAINING

MUSCLE GROUP	EXERCISE	RESISTANCE BAND	REPS

NUMBERS OF CIRCUITS -	
REST BETWEEN CIRCUITS -	

SUPERSETS				
SUPERSET	EXERCISES	RESISTANCE BAND	REPS	SETS
#1				
#2				
#3				
#4				
#5				
#6				
#7				

The Exercises

Chest Exercises

Chest press anchor at the top

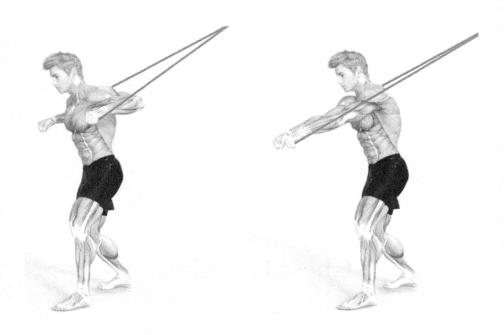

Set up - An exercise designed to hit the chest muscles along with the triceps muscles (upper, rear arms). Select a resistance band for your current fitness level and either use the door anchor at the top of the door or loop the band around a stable fixing above head height. You can attach stirrups as shown in the picture or simply grip the ends of the band in your fists.

Start position – Hold the ends of the band or the stirrups in your fists with your palms facing down. Step forward with one foot to form a stable base. Keep your back flat, abs engaged, and look forward. Position yourself so you feel slight tension in the band when your arms are parallel with the floor and your elbows are back.

Movement – As you exhale, slowly and under control, push your fists forward and slightly down. As you do this, you can choose to gradually bring each hand into the centre line of your body to finish with your thumbs nearly touching to get an extra contraction. You should stop just before your elbows lock. Once you reach this point, inhale while returning to the start position. This completes one rep.

Chest press with door anchor at the bottom

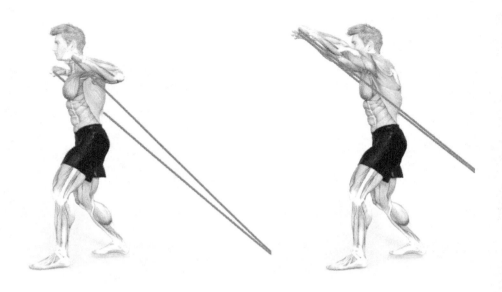

Set up - This is a compound movement to hit the upper chest. Thread the exercise band through the door anchor and attach it at the bottom of a door. Ensure that the loop of the door anchor is placed in the middle of the exercise band. Attach the stirrups to each end of the band.

Start position – Take a grip of the stirrups so your palms are facing down. Your fists should be in line with your upper chest and elbows bent. Step forward with one foot and keep your knees slightly bent for stability. Keep your back flat, abs engaged, feet flat on the floor and look forward.

Movement – As you exhale, slowly and under control, push your fists forward and slightly upwards. As you do this, you can choose to gradually bring each hand into the centre line of your body to finish with your thumbs nearly touching to get an extra contraction. You should stop just before your elbows lock. Once you reach this point, inhale while returning to the start position.

Chest press without door anchor

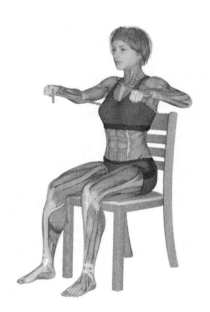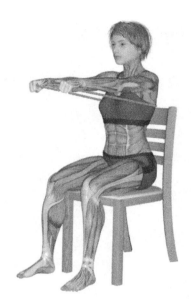

Set up - An exercise designed to hit the chest muscles along with the triceps muscles (upper, rear arms). Sit on a sturdy chair, select a resistance band for your current fitness level and loop this around your body or use the door anchor in the side of a door so the anchor point is in line with your shoulder blades when sitting. Grip the ends of the band in your fists so that your palms are facing inwards.

Start position – Hold the ends of the band in your fists with your palms facing downwards. Sit with your back flat, abs engaged, feet flat on the floor and looking forward. Keep your elbows close to your sides and push them back slightly. You should now adjust your grip on the band at this point so that you feel slight tension.

Movement – As you exhale, slowly and under control, push your fists forward directly in front of you. As you do this, you can choose to gradually bring each hand into the centre line of your body to finish with your thumbs nearly touching to get an extra contraction. You should stop just before your elbows lock. Once you reach this point, inhale while returning to the start position. This completes one rep.

Flyes with door anchor at the top

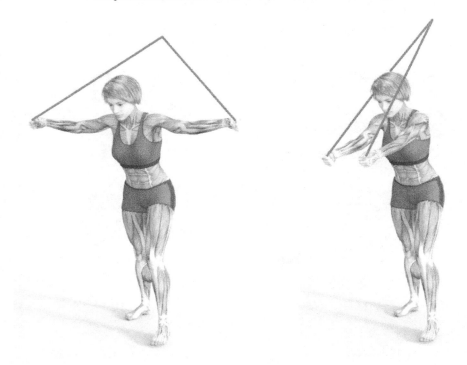

Set up – An isolation exercise to target the lower chest muscles. Loop an exercise band through the door anchor and attach the anchor to the top of a door. Attach the stirrups (optional) and grip the ends of the band, palms facing inwards.

Start position – Stand with one foot in front of the other, knees slightly bent. Engage your core and hinge at the hip slightly. Lift your arms so they are out to your sides and about parallel with the floor, elbows slightly bent. At this point, you may need to shift your position forward to create tension on the band.

Movement – As you exhale, slowly and under control, pull your fists towards your body's centre line and slightly down. Your elbows should remain as per the start position. Once at the top of movement, as you inhale, return to the start position. This completes one rep.

Flyes with door anchor at the bottom

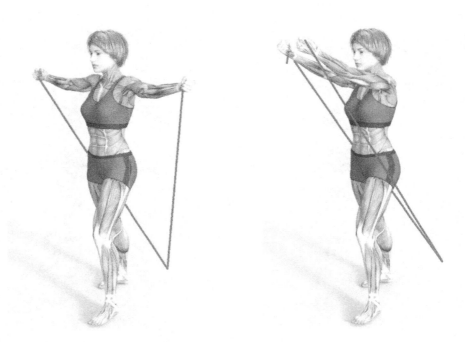

Set up - An isolation exercise designed to hit the upper chest muscles. Select a resistance band for your current fitness level and attach the door anchor at the bottom of a door. Grip the stirrups or the end of the band in your fists so that your palms are facing inwards.

Start position – Hold the ends of the band in your fists with your palms facing inwards. Extend your arms to so they are straight, but just before your elbows lock, your arms should be parallel to the ground and out to your sides. Step forward with one foot to form a stable base. Keep your back flat, abs engaged, and look forward. Position yourself so you feel slight tension on the band and only to where you feel a slight stretch through your chest muscles.

Movement – As you exhale, slowly and under control, pull your fists towards your midline and slightly upwards. When you reach the midline and your hands are about to touch in front of you, slowly return to the start position while inhaling. This completes one rep. Your elbow joint should remain in a fixed position throughout this movement as not to dilute the workload from the chest muscles.

Back Exercises

Lat pulldowns with door anchor at the top

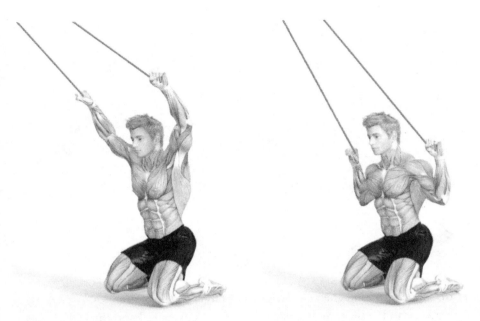

Set up - An exercise designed to hit the back muscles. Select a resistance band for your current fitness level and either use the door anchor at the top of the door or loop the band around a stable fixing above head height. You can attach stirrups as shown in the picture or simply grip the ends of the band in your fists.

Start position – Grip the stirrups or the end of the band so that your palms are facing forwards. Kneel on the floor. Extend your arms to so they are above your head but just before your elbows lock. At this point, adjust your grip on the band if you can't feel slight tension. Keep your back flat, abs engaged, and look forward.

Movement – As you exhale, slowly and under control, pull your fists down and elbows back and down. You should also push your chest slightly forward to add more value to the working back muscles. When your fists are just above shoulder height, this is the top of the movement and the point where you inhale and slowly return to the start position. This completes one rep.

Bent over rows with door anchor

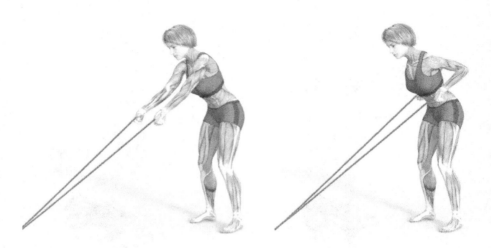

Set up – A compound exercise designed to target the back muscles. Attach the door anchor to the bottom of a door and loop an exercise band through. You can use the hand stirrups or simply grip each end of the band.

Start position – Hold the ends of the band in your fists with your palms facing inwards. Keep your back flat, abs engaged and feet about hip width apart. Stand straight and hinge at the hips slightly. Extend your arms out in front of you until you have a small bend in the elbows. At this point, you may need to shift your feet position away from the door to create tension on the band.

Movement – As you exhale, pull your fists towards your navel. Your elbows should graze the sides of your body as they pass. Once your fists are in line with your sides, you have reached the top of movement. As you inhale, return to the start position.

Seated row with door anchor

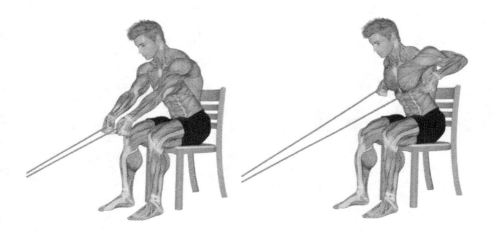

Set up – A compound exercise designed to target the back muscles. Attach the door anchor to the bottom of a door and loop an exercise band through. You can use the hand stirrups or simply grip each end of the band. Set up a chair in front of the door anchor at a distance that will allow tension of the band when gripped.

Start position – Sit on the chair whilst holding the ends of the band. Keep your back flat, abs engaged and feet about hip width apart. Hinge at the hips slightly. Hold the ends of the band in your fists with your palms facing inwards. Extend your arms out in front of you until you have a small bend in the elbows.

Movement – As you exhale, pull your fists towards your navel. Your elbows should graze the sides of your body as they pass. Once your fists are in line with your sides, you have reached the top of movement. As you inhale, return to the start position.

Bent over rows with band under feet

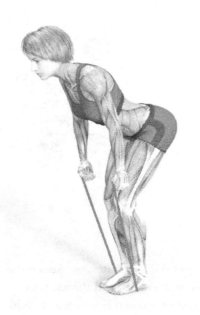 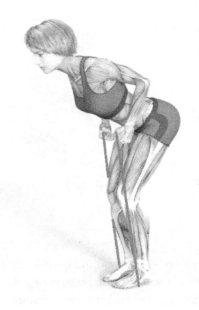

Set up – A compound exercise designed to target the back muscles. Select a resistance band for your current fitness level, place it on the floor and step onto it with both feet, ensuring that there are even lengths on either side to work with. You can attach stirrups or simply grip the ends of the band in your fists.

Start position – Grip the stirrups or the end of the band so that your palms are facing inwards, keep your arms extended but elbows slightly bent. Keep your back flat, abs engaged and look forward. Hold this position before hinging at your hips to lean forward slightly. At this point, adjust your grip on the band if you can't feel slight tension.

Movement – As you exhale, slowly and under control, pull your fists up towards your belly button, ensuring that your elbows do not flare out too much. You should also push your chest slightly forward to add more value to the working back muscles. When your fists are at your sides, this is the top of the movement and the point where you inhale and slowly return to the start position. This completes one rep. A point to note here is that if you choose to bring your fists closer to your midline, you will focus more on the inner back muscles and vice versa.

Pullovers

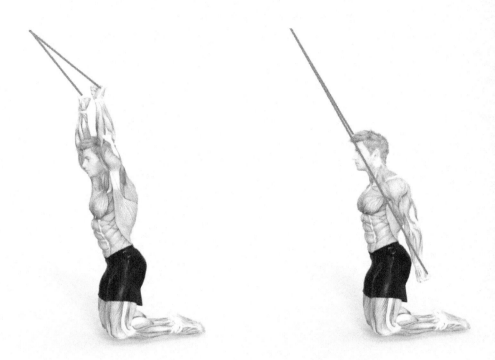

Set up – An isolation exercise to target the back muscles. Loop a resistance band through the door anchor and secure at the top of a door. Hand stirrups are optional on this exercise, but due to the nature of this exercise, it may be hard to start with tension on the band with the stirrups. It may be that you have to grip the band closer to the middle to ensure tension throughout the movement.

Start position – Grip the stirrups or the ends of the band. Kneel on the floor close to the door. Engage your core and glutes and with a flat back, lift your arms so they are above your head. They should be straight but with a slight bend in the elbows. Your palms should face forward.

Movement – As you exhale, slowly lower your straight arms to bring your fists just past your glutes. As you do so, push your chest forward and shoulders back. The only joints that should move in this exercise are your shoulders. Once at the top of movement, as you inhale, return to the start position.

*** At the top of movement, some trainers will push their hips forwards to increase the range of movement and engage the lower back, but this is for those who are comfortable with the exercise.

Seated rows on chair

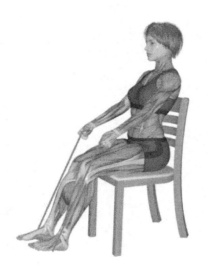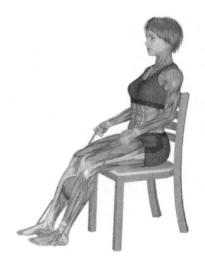

Set up – A compound exercise designed to target the back muscles. Select a resistance band for your current fitness level, sit on a sturdy chair and loop the band around both feet, ensuring that there are even lengths on either side to work with. You can attach stirrups or simply grip the ends of the band in your fists.

Start position – Grip the stirrups or the end of the band so that your palms are facing inwards keep your arms extended but elbows slightly bent. Keep your back flat, abs engaged, and look forward. Plant your heals into the floor at about a 45-degree angle from the seat. At this point, adjust your grip on the band if you can't feel slight tension.

Movement – As you exhale, slowly and under control, pull your fists up towards your belly button, ensuring that your elbows do not flare out too much. You should also push your chest slightly forward to add more value to the working back muscles. When your fists are at your sides, this is the top of the movement and the point where you inhale and slowly return to the start position. This completes one rep. A point to note here is that if you choose to bring your fists closer to your midline, you will focus more on the inner back muscles and vice versa.

The Superhero

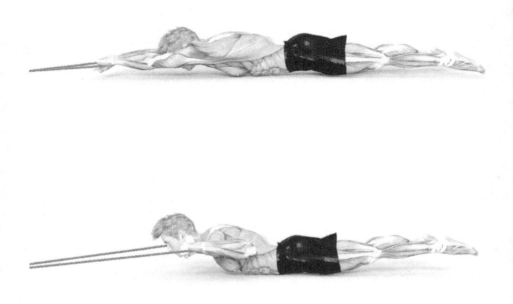

Set up – A compound exercise designed to target the back muscles. Select a resistance band for your current fitness level and attach stirrups (optional). Attach the band to the door anchor and secure at the bottom of a door. Position yourself so your body is flat on the floor, face down, and arms outstretched above your head. You should set up at this position so when you grip the band, there is already tension.

Start position – Grip the ends of the band so your palms are facing the floor. Your back should be flat, abs and glutes engaged and tops of feet should be in contact with the floor. Although your arms are outstretched, you should still have a slight bend in the elbows.

Movement – As you exhale, pull your fists towards the outside of your shoulders, keeping your elbows in line with the sides of your body. As you make this movement, slightly lift your head to increase the contraction. Once your fists are in line with the tops of your shoulders, you have reached the top of movement, at this point, as you exhale, return to the start position. This completes one rep.

*** Note that this is a fairly advanced movement and there is an option to also lift your feet slightly off the floor to add hyperextension to your lower back, but this is only advised for more advanced trainers.

Deadlift

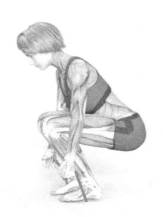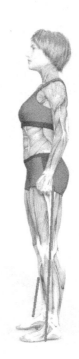

Set up – A compound exercise for the back and legs. Select a resistance band, place it on the floor and stand in the middle, feet about shoulder width apart. Make sure you have even lengths on either side of your feet.

Start position – Grip the ends of the band, palms facing inwards and close to your shins. Engage your core, keep your back flat, and position yourself in a squat. The deeper the squat position, the more effect this exercise will have on the legs. When in this position, ensure that you already have a bit of tension in the band.

Movement – As you exhale, push through the middle of your feet to straighten your knees. Keep your back flat, shoulder muscles engaged and elbows locked in a slightly bent position. Once at the top of movement, pause before slowly returning to the start position. This completes one rep.

60

*** Deadlift is an advanced exercise, and it should not be attempted unless you can perform bodyweight squats with comfort.

Leg Exercises

Single leg abduction

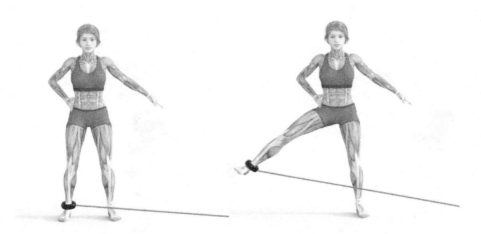

Set up – An isolation exercise for the outer, upper leg muscles. Attach an exercise band to the door anchor and secure at the bottom of a door. Attach an ankle strap to the opposite end of the band and secure the ankle strap to the ankle of the working leg. Position yourself so that there is tension on the band when standing straight.

Start position – Stand with your feet shoulder width apart, knees slightly bent. Keep a flat back and engage your abs and glutes. Hand and arm position is optional, but some prefer to have both hands out for balance, both hands on the hips or a combination of both.

Movement – As you exhale, lift your leg out to the side, working against the resistance of the band. You should maintain torso alignment as per the start position. The working leg should move directly out and not track forwards or backwards. Once at the top of movement, reverse the process as you inhale. Once you have completed your target reps on this leg, switch legs and repeat.

Kick backs

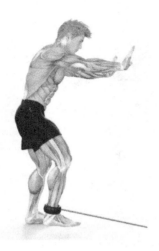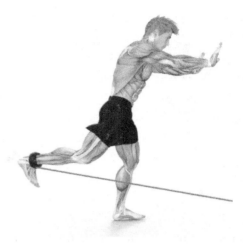

Set up – An isolation exercise for the glutes. Attach the ankle strap to the working ankle and the other end of the band to the door anchor and secure at the bottom of a door. Depending on the length of the band, you may need to double the band over (making it half the length) or stand further away from the door. It's possible to place a solid object, such as a chair, between you and the door. The chair can be used to lean on too.

Start position – Stand with your feet about hip width apart, bend at the knees slightly and engage your core. Hinge at the hips to take the weight of your upper body against the door or chair. Keep your back flat whilst you do this. Once in this position, transfer your body weight to your stabilising foot as you bend the knee of your working leg slightly to bring your foot slightly off the floor.

Movement – As you exhale, and whilst maintaining your body alignment, extend your leg backwards as you engage your working glute. Your knee should remain as per the start position. Once at the top of movement, as you inhale, reverse the process. Once you have completed your target number of reps, repeat on the opposite leg.

*** This exercise might take some practice for beginners to develop a mind muscle connection, but when this is achieved, the movement can be more exaggerated, meaning you can add a forward leaning movement with your upper body during each rep to get a deeper contraction in the glutes.

Leg lifts

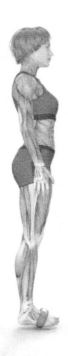 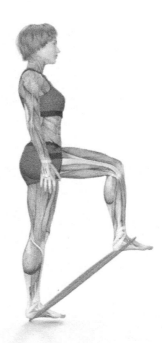

Set up - An exercise designed to hit the upper leg muscles to develop stability. Select a resistance band for your current fitness level. You can use a loop exercise band or create a loop if you have a band with attachments by hooking the ends together. As this is a small movement, you will need a small band. This can be created by forming a figure eight with the looped band and folding together. If you do this, it's important to note that the band will have double the resistance.

Start position – Place the loop on the floor around your feet, which should be about shoulder width apart. Stand up straight, keep your back flat, abs engaged, and look forward. Your knees should not be locked, they should be slightly bent, and your quads should be engaged. The loop band should be at a slight tension in this position.

Movement – As you exhale, slowly and under control, pull one leg up until your quad is parallel with the floor. The sole of your foot should also be parallel with the floor or toes slightly pointing up to add extra value to the exercise. If you have trouble with balancing, put your arms out to your sides or use a stable abject to steady yourself. This is the top of the movement and the point where you inhale and slowly return to the start position. A point to note here is that if you need to steady yourself, you should not use this to weight bear. This completes one rep.

Resistance band squats

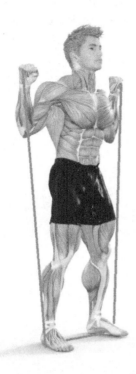
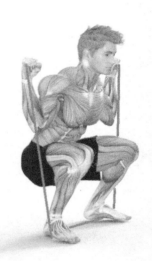

Set up - An exercise designed to hit the upper leg muscles. Select a resistance band for your current fitness level. You can use a big loop band or an exercise band with stirrup attachments.

Start position – Place the exercise band on the floor and stand on it with both feet so that they are about shoulder width apart, toes are pointing out slightly and that there are even lengths of exercise band on either side. Pick up the stirrups so that your palms are facing forwards and in line with your chin, stand up straight, keep your back flat, abs engaged, and look forward. Your knees should not be locked, they should be slightly bent, and your quads should be engaged.

Movement – As you inhale, slowly and under control, squat down until your quads are parallel with the floor, ensuring that you maintain a flat back, you maintain the position of your hands and feet. Once you hit this position, you are at the top of the movement and, as you exhale, slowly return to the start position. This completes one rep.

Lunges

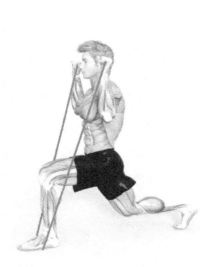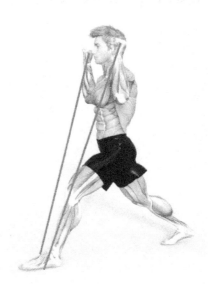

Set up – An exercise designed to target the upper leg muscles. Select an exercise band that allows you to train inside your target workload. This exercise can be performed with or without the hand stirrups.

Start position – Place your leading foot on the middle of the resistance band, ensuring you have even lengths on either side. Grip the hand stirrups or ends of the band, position your arms so your fists are in line with the sides of your head and your palms facing forward. Kneel down on the floor, ensuring your leading leg forms a right angle at the knee from your hamstring to your calf and the quad of your trailing leg is in line with your upper body. Your upper body should be straight, with your core engaged. Finally, push through your toes to lift your knee off the floor slightly.

Movement – As you exhale, push through the middle of your leading foot to straighten your legs. Ensure that at the top of movement that you do not lock your knees, there should always be a slight bend in the knee. Maintain an engaged core and flat back throughout the movement. Once you reach the top of movement, as you inhale, return to the start position. Once you have completed a set, switch legs and repeat.

*** This is an advanced exercise and may take some practice and experimentation to perfect. The start position is important on this one, especially the position of the leading leg. If your foot is too far forward or backward, it can put undue strain on the knee joint.

Seated calf raises

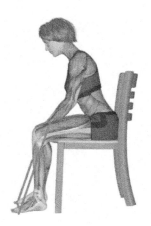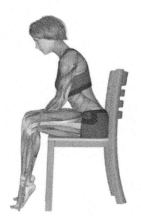

Set up - An exercise designed to hit the lower leg muscles. Select a resistance band for your current fitness level. You can use a loop band or an exercise band with or without stirrup attachments.

Start position – Sit on a chair with your feet flat to the floor. Take the exercise band in both hands, hinge forward at the hips so the band runs across the top of your quads, just above your knees. Secure the band underneath your toes, then push your fists forward slightly between your knees.

Movement – As you exhale, push through the balls of your feet to raise your knees. Continue until your calves are at maximum contraction. Once at the top of movement, as you inhale, return to the start position. This completes one rep. Your hands should remain in the start position throughout the movement.

Arm Exercises

Supination curls with door anchor

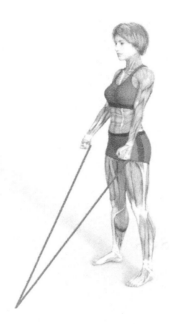 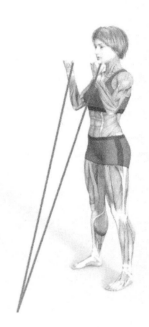

Set up - This is an exercise to target both heads of the biceps. Loop the band through the door anchor and secure the anchor at the bottom of a door. It's best not to attach the hand stirrups in this exercise, so grip the ends of the band in your fists, palms facing inwards.

Start position – Stand with your knees slightly bent, back flat and core engaged. Your feet should be about shoulder width apart. With your arms straight, fists facing inwards, position yourself so there is tension in the band by stepping away from the door.

Movement – As you exhale, bend your elbows to bring your fists towards your shoulders. As you progress through this movement, slowly twist your palms. When you reach maximum contraction of your biceps, your palms should face your shoulders. Once at the top of movement, as you inhale, return to the start position. This completes one rep.

Drag curl

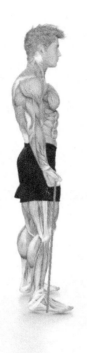 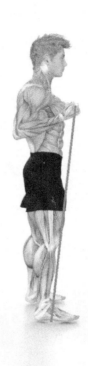

Set up – This is an exercise for the biceps. Select an exercise band that allows you to perform in your target work zone, hand stirrups are optional. Stand on the exercise band so you have even lengths either side of your feet with your feet about shoulder width apart.

Start position – Take hold of the ends of the band or the stirrups and stand up straight with your arms by your sides, palms facing forward. Your arms should be straight but elbows should not be locked, so keep a slight bend in them. Engage your core and keep your back flat.

Movement – As you exhale, drag your fists upwards, keeping them close to your body. This will force your elbows up and backwards. Once at maximum contraction, as you inhale, return to the start position. This completes one rep.

*** Not that this is a smaller movement that other types of bicep curl and it may take some practice before getting the right feel for the movement. It's common to feel the need to lean forward during this exercise, but you should maintain an upright position throughout the movement.

Standing bicep curls

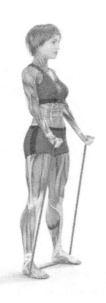 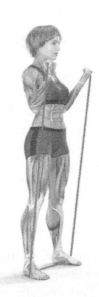

Set up - An exercise designed to hit the upper front arm muscles. Select a resistance band for your current fitness level. You can use an exercise band with stirrup attachments or without.

Start position – Place the exercise band on the floor and stand on it with one foot. There should be even lengths of exercise band on either side. Your rear foot should be planted to steady yourself and your knees should be slightly bent. Pick up the stirrups so that your palms are facing forwards and take the strain of the band. Your elbows should be slightly bent, stand up straight, keep your back flat, abs engaged, and look forward.

Movement – As you exhale, slowly and under control, bring your fists up towards your front shoulder. Ensure that your elbows are stationary; you should feel this working your biceps. Once you are at the top of the movement as you inhale, slowly return to the start position. This completes one rep.

Preacher curl

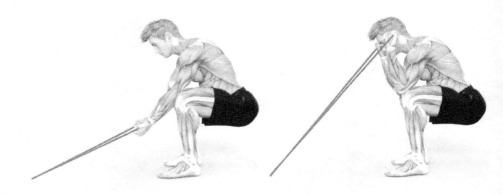

Set up – This is an isolation exercise for the biceps. Loop an exercise band through the door anchor and attach at the bottom of a door. Attaching the hand stirrups is preferable, but this can be performed without them.

Start position – Grip the hand stirrups and adopt a squat position a few steps back from the door. Bring your upper, rear arms to your front and rest on your knees them so your elbows are just in front of your knees. Straighten your arms until there is only a slight bend in your elbows, palms should face upwards. If there is no tension in the band at this point, reposition yourself further away from the door.

Movement – As you exhale, bend at your elbows to bring your fists towards the sides of your head. Your wrists should not twist and should remain as per the start position. Once you have reached the top of movement, as you inhale, return to the start position under control. This completes one rep.

*** If you struggle to hold a static squat position, this exercise is possible to perform whilst seated on a low chair or exercise step

Overhead tricep extensions

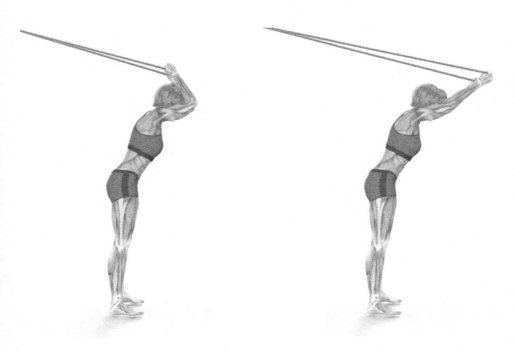

Set up - An exercise designed to hit the upper, rear arm muscles. Select a resistance band for your current fitness level and either use the door anchor at the top of the door or loop the band around a stable fixing about head height. It's best to use an exercise band without the stirrups for this exercise. Simply grip the ends of the band in your fists.

Start position – Grip the stirrups or the end of the band so that your palms are facing inwards. Stand with your back towards the anchor point. Lift your lower arms so they are at around 45 degrees to the floor. Let the tension of the band pull your lower arms back behind your head. Adjust your grip on the band if you can't feel slight tension or take a step forward. Keep your back flat, abs engaged and look forward and slightly lean forward, hinging at your hips. You can place one foot in front of the other to form a stable base if necessary.

Movement – As you exhale, slowly and under control, bring your upper arms out in front of you to the point just before your elbows lock, this is the top of the movement and the point where you inhale and slowly return to the start position. It's important to note that your upper arms should remain fixed in this position throughout the set. This completes one rep. You should feel this working in your upper rear arms.

Standing tricep kickbacks

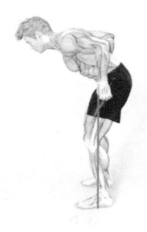 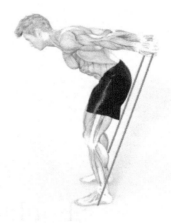

Set up - An exercise designed to hit the upper, rear arm muscles. Select a resistance band for your current fitness level and either attach stirrups to either end or simply grip the ends of the band in your fists. Stirrups are recommended for this exercise.

Start position – Place the exercise band on the floor and stand on it with both feet so that they are about shoulder width apart, toes are pointing out slightly and that there are even lengths of exercise band on either side. Pick up the stirrups so that your palms are facing forward. Keep your back flat, abs engaged and look forward. Your knees should not be locked, they should be slightly bent, and your quads should be engaged. Hinge at the hips so your upper body is at a 45-degree angle with the floor. Pull your upper arms up so they are parallel to the floor.

Movement – As you exhale, slowly and under control, bring your lower arms up to the point just before your elbows lock. This is the top of the movement and the point where you inhale and slowly return to the start position. It's important to note that your upper arms should remain fixed in this position throughout the set. This completes one rep. You should feel this working in your upper rear arms.

Shoulder Exercises

Lateral raises band under feet

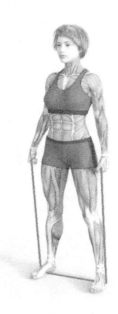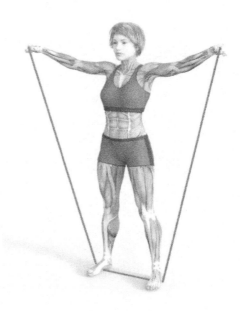

Set up - An exercise designed to hit the mid shoulder muscles. Select a resistance band for your current fitness level and either attach stirrups to either end or simply grip the ends of the band in your fists. Stirrups are recommended for this exercise.

Start position – Place the exercise band on the floor and stand on it with both feet so that they are close together, toes are pointing out slightly and that there are even lengths of exercise band on either side. Pick up the stirrups so that your palms are facing inwards. Your arms should be by your sides and elbows, slightly bent. Keep your back flat, abs engaged, and look forward. Your knees should not be locked, they should be slightly bent, and your quads should be engaged. Pull your upper arms up so they are parallel to the floor.

Movement – As you exhale, slowly and under control, bring your arms up until they are just above parallel with the floor. This is the top of the movement and the point where you inhale and slowly return to the start position. It's important to note that your elbows should remain fixed throughout the set. This completes one rep. You should feel this working your mid shoulder muscles.

Front raises

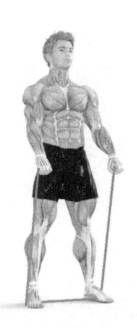 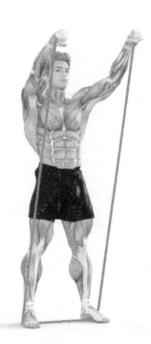

Set up - This is an isolation exercise for the front deltoids. Select a band that fits with your target workload, place it on the floor and step onto the middle, feet about shoulder width apart, ensuring there are even lengths on either side of your feet. Attach the hand stirrups and grip them with your palms facing towards your thighs.

Start position – Engage your core, keep your back flat, knees slightly bent and head in a neutral position. Ensure you have a slight bend in your elbows, but arms straight. Lift your arms in front of you slightly to add a small amount of tension to the band.

Movement – As you exhale, lift your arms by rotating your shoulders. Your elbows and wrists should remain as per the start position. Continue the movement until your arms are above parallel to the floor. Your arms should also not track inwards or outwards. As you inhale, slowly return to the start position. This completes one rep.

Reverse flyes

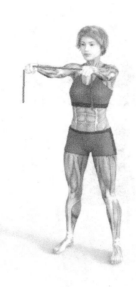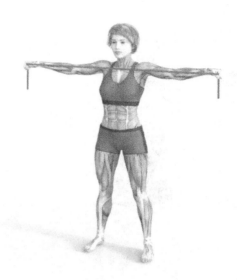

Set up - An exercise designed to hit the rear shoulder muscles. Select a resistance band for your current fitness level. You can either use a loop band or create a loop by linking the ends of a straight band.

Start position - Pick up the band and hold it out in front of you so that your palms are facing downwards and your arms are extended with a slight bend in the elbows and parallel with the floor. Keep your back flat, abs engaged and look forward. Your knees should not be locked, they should be slightly bent, and your quads should be engaged.

Movement – As you exhale, slowly and under control, bring your fists out to your sides until they are almost in line with your chest. Your elbows should remain fixed and arms should remain parallel to the floor throughout the movement. This is the top of the movement and the point where you inhale and slowly return to the start position. This completes one rep. You should feel this working your rear shoulder muscles.

Seated shoulder press

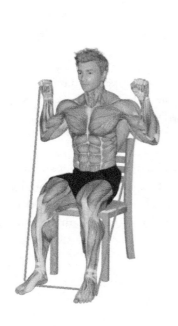 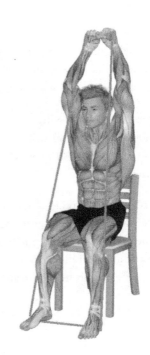

Set up - An exercise designed to hit all three heads of the shoulder muscles. Select a resistance band for your current fitness level and either attach stirrups to either end or simply grip the ends of the band in your fists. Stirrups are recommended for this exercise.

Start position – Sit on a sturdy chair or bench with the exercise band running underneath your glutes, making sure that there are even lengths of exercise band either side. Pick up the stirrups so that your palms are facing forwards and in line with your chin. Keep your back flat, abs engaged and look forward.

Movement – As you exhale, slowly and under control, bring your arms up and directly above your head, ensuring not to lock out your elbows. This is the top of the movement and the point where you inhale and slowly return to the start position. This completes one rep. You should feel this working your shoulder muscles.

Abdominal exercises

Although this is a guide to working out with exercise bands, it is also a guide to effective resistance training with a focus on full body workouts. This is why I have chosen to include some abdominal exercises.

If you are training with a resistance routine, and you are performing the exercises with good form, you will be engaging your abdominal muscles through every rep of every set for all the exercise choices. This promotes core strength and good posture.

Exercises that directly target the abdominals can be used to further strengthen these muscles. When targeting the abs with specific exercises, they should always be the last exercise in your training session. This is because they are used as support and stabilisation for all other exercises and you don't want them to be fatigued early on in your training session.

Resistance band crunch

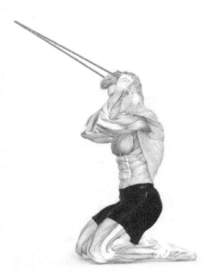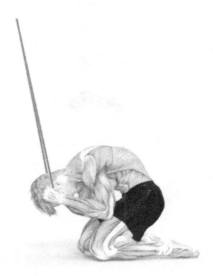

Set up - An exercise designed to target the abdominal muscles. Loop a resistance band through the door anchor and attach at the top of a door. It's best not to attach the stirrups for this exercise and grip the ends instead. Depending on your height, you may want to grip the band closet to the middle and wrap the excess around your hands.

Start position – Kneel on the floor close to the door. Your shins and tops of your feet should be in contact with the ground. Lift your arms so your fists are in contact with the side of your head, palms facing inwards. At this point you can choose to sit right back onto the backs of your legs or keep your upper legs at a wider angle from them. Engage your core and glutes.

Movement – As you exhale, contract your abs by bending through the middle of your back. Keep your fists and arms fixed in the start position to use the position of your elbows as a gauge – For more emphasis on the upper abdominals, aim for your elbows to hit your quads. For more emphasis on your lower abs, aim for your elbows to hit nearer your knees. Once at the top of movement, as you inhale, return to the start position.

Swiss ball crunches

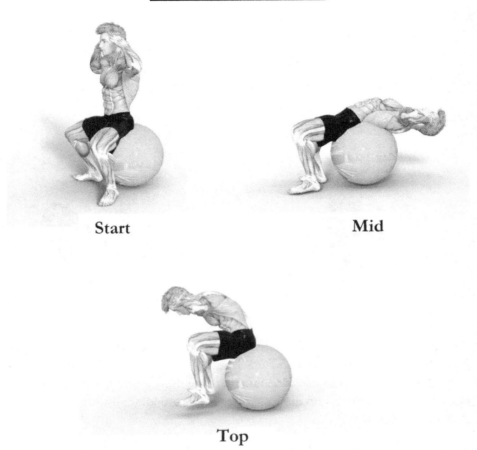

Start

Mid

Top

Set up - An exercise designed to hit the abdominal muscles. An exercise ball is perfect for this movement and a valuable piece of home workout equipment.

Start position – Sit on the exercise ball, keep your back flat, abs engaged, and look forward as you would for shoulder press. Plant your feet on the floor just past shoulder width apart to steady yourself. Once you are stable, slowly walk your feet forward while leaning backward, allowing the ball to roll into the small of your back. Place your fingers on the side of your head.

Movement – As you exhale, slowly and under control, raise your upper body until it reaches a 45-degree angle to the floor by hinging at the hips. This is the top of the movement and the point where you inhale and slowly return to the start position. This completes one rep. You should feel this working your abdominal muscles. A point to note here is that the closer together you can bring your feet, the more challenging this exercise will become, as you will use more stabiliser muscles for stability.

Lower abdominal crunch

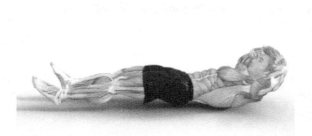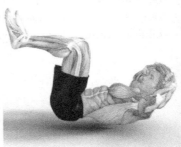

Set up - An exercise designed to hit the abdominal muscles with a stronger focus on the lower section. This is a body weight exercise that does not require any equipment.

Start position – Lie on the floor, keep your back flat, abs engaged, and lift your head and shoulders slightly to engage your abdominals. Place your fingers on your temples. Straighten your legs, ensuring you have a slight bend through the knees. Finally, raise your heels slightly so they are off the floor. This will further engage your abs.

Movement – As you exhale, slowly and under control, bring your upper legs towards your body. This is the top of the movement and the point where you inhale and slowly return to the start position. This completes one rep. You should feel this working your lower abdominal muscles. A point to note here is that on returning to the start position, always keep your heels off the floor. This will keep your abs engaged throughout the set.

Elevated leg crunch

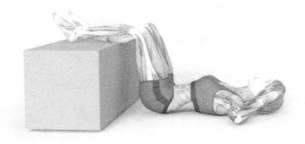

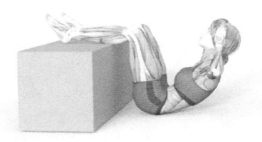

Set up - An exercise designed to hit the abdominal muscles with a stronger focus on the upper section. This is a body weight exercise, but some means of elevation is required. You can use a chair, sofa, or any other object that will support your lower legs at a right angle to the floor. Advanced trainers can do this exercise without equipment.

Start position – position yourself on the floor so you can rest your lower legs on your chosen support at a right angle to the floor. Lay flat on your back, putting your fingers on the side of your head. Finally, raise your head and shoulders off the floor slightly to engage your abdominal muscles.

Movement – As you exhale, slowly and under control, bring your upper body towards your legs. This is the top of the movement and the point where you inhale and slowly return to the start position. This completes one rep. You should feel this working your abdominal muscles. A point to note here is that on returning to the start position, always keep your head and shoulders off the floor. This will keep your abs engaged throughout the set.

Multi movement exercises

The exercise movements listed until now have been focused on a single muscle group. This is an excellent way to train with resistance, but there are more ways to use these movements as you become a more advanced trainer and start looking for more challenging workouts.

In this small section, we will look at a few movements that merge several exercises together to hit several large muscle groups in a single movement.

As these exercises choices use multiple large muscle groups to perform a single rep, they will be far more demanding on the body, which will lead to increased stamina, muscle strength, fat burning and cardio fitness. It's because of this that exercise form when performing these movements should be even more scrutinised.

If you are a beginner or not experienced with resistance band training, these exercises should be something that you work up to. They are not really advised for newer trainers. If, however, you feel that this is the type of training that you really want to do, make sure that you practise and perfect the movement before adding it to your workouts.

If you decide to use this type of exercise, you can fit them in anywhere in your workout, but keep in mind that these are big movements and they will lead to fatigue a lot quicker than the other exercises listed.

Squat with row

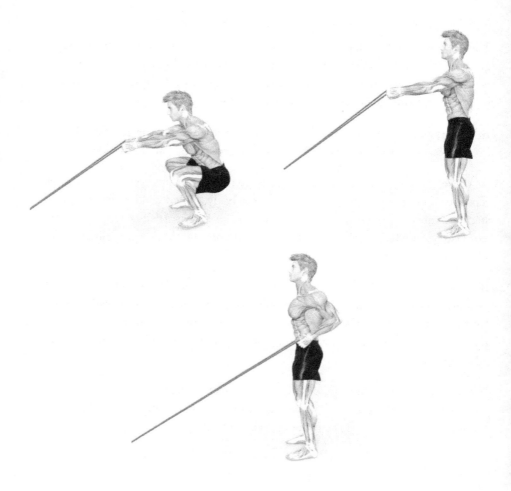

Set up - An exercise designed to hit the legs and back muscles. Select a resistance band for your current fitness level. You can attach stirrups or simply grip the ends of the band in your fists. This exercise can be done with a single-handed grip using a door anchor and loop band or double handed with the stirrups and door anchor attached at the bottom of the door.

Start position – Grip the stirrups or the end of the band so that your palms are facing inwards. Keep your arms extended but elbows slightly bent and hands in line with your lower abdomen. Keep your back flat, abs engaged, and look forward. Step away from the door until the resistance band is slightly under tension and you are standing up straight, as per the starting position for squats.

Movement – As you inhale, slowly and under control, squat down so your quads are parallel with the floor, arms should still be extended in front of you at this point. As you exhale, return to the start position, but as you do so, bring your fists in towards your lower abdomen as if you were performing a row. This completes one rep. A point to note here is that exercise form with the squat and the row should never be sacrificed in order to perform more reps. This is an advanced exercise.

Deadlift and row

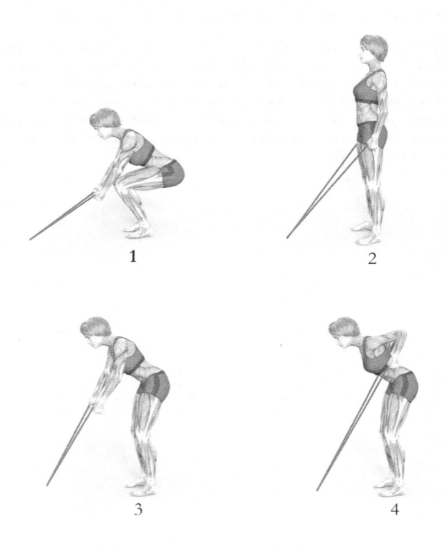

1

2

3

4

Set up - An exercise designed to hit the legs and back muscles. Select a resistance band for your current fitness level. You can attach stirrups or simply grip the ends of the band in your fists. This exercise can be done with a single handed grip using a door anchor and loop band or double handed with the stirrups and door anchor attached at the bottom of the door.

Start position – Grip the stirrups or the end of the band so that your palms are facing inwards. Keep your arms extended but elbows slightly bent and hands in line with your lower abdomen. Keep your back flat, abs engaged. Hinge at the waist until your upper body is just above parallel with the floor. You may need to shuffle away from the door until the resistance band is slightly under tension. Your knees should be slightly bent to put you into a half squat position. Your back should always be flat.

Movement – As you exhale, slowly, under control and in one smooth movement hinge at the waist and straighten your legs to bring you into an upright position whilst also pulling your fists toward your outer thighs. Once in this position (2), hinge at the hips and move your arms away from your body slightly (position 3). From here, pull your fists into your lower abdomen whilst pulling your shoulders backwards (position 4). This completes one rep.

*** A point to note here is that if you are performing this exercise with a single hand grip, you should take extra care not to twist. With practice, this will become a single movement. This is an advanced exercise.

Squat with shoulder press

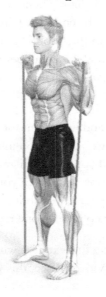

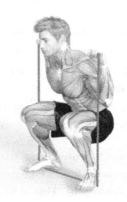

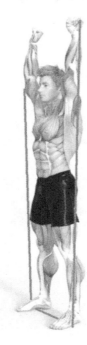

Set up - An exercise designed to hit the legs and shoulder muscles. Select a resistance band for your current fitness level. You can either attach stirrups or use a large loop band. This exercise is performed using bodyweight as an anchor.

Start position – Place the exercise band on the floor and stand on it with both feet so that they are about shoulder width apart, toes are pointing out slightly and that there are even lengths of exercise band on either side. Pick up the stirrups so that your palms are facing forwards and in line with your chin, stand up straight, keep your back flat, abs engaged, and look forward. Your knees should not be locked, they should be slightly bent, and your quads should be engaged.

Movement – As you inhale, slowly and under control, squat down until your quads are parallel with the floor, ensuring that you maintain a flat back, you maintain the position of your hands and feet. Once you hit this position, as you exhale, slowly return through the start position to perform a shoulder press. When performing the shoulder press, bring your arms up and directly above your head, ensuring not to lock out your elbows. Once at the top of this movement, slowly return to the start position. This completes one rep. A point to note here is that the resistance level of your exercise band is dictated by your ability to shoulder press.

Upgrade your workout?

Resistance bands and resistance band training are extremely versatile. The more you train with these fantastic pieces of exercise equipment, and the more experienced you get, the more ways you will discover of using them.

I highly recommend that you explore different training methods and experiment with different exercises, as you may find some interesting ways of training that you enjoy and also align with your goals.

If you have created your own plan using the templates that I've provided, I want to outline a few more options for you to add variation, maybe give you some inspiration and to ultimately show you that there is a lot that you can do to progress, add variation or give yourself more of a challenge.

Add exercises

Adding exercises to your workout will give you a longer training session, along with more variety. If you are thinking of adding exercises, you can consider the type of exercise. Compound exercises use more energy to perform compared to isolation exercises. So a shoulder press will burn more calories and use more muscle groups to perform than lateral raises, so if your goal is fat burning and general muscle tone, shoulder press will be your best choice if you were looking to add a shoulder exercise.

You may also have identified a weakness in a certain muscle group and want to turn those weaknesses into strengths. It's possible to do this by adding extra exercises in for that muscle group. You can even replace exercises that target muscle groups you don't need as much work on with these. This way, you keep the training volume as it is but push the focus towards a slightly different goal.

Add resistance

More resistance means more development, but it is so important that you never sacrifice exercise form for more resistance! If you are exercising in good form and a resistance level that challenges you, you are doing well.

There are two ways to add resistance to your workouts. You can simply change the exercise band that you have been working with to the next level of resistance band tension or you can stack the bands. Stacking exercise bands is an excellent way to increase resistance level. I own several full sets of exercise bands and often use the heaviest resistance band from each set to perform big exercises such as squats.

Stacking bands like this can give you a very steep curve of resistance progression, which is great for bodybuilders or strength trainers, but it can also give a small increment increase, too. If you find yourself in a situation where one tension of exercise band is not challenging enough but the next tension in your set is too challenging, you can stack several of the lower resistance bands in the set together.

Add sets

Adding sets is a simple way to upgrade your workout. You can choose to add an extra set to all exercises in your session, or just a few. If you are challenging yourself with the reps in each set, a solid amount of sets to work with is between 3 and 5. Extra sets can be added for all training methods but depending on your choice here, you may want to consider the exercise choices and methods along with your current fitness levels. Adding an extra set of bicep curls to your single exercise routine will have a lot less impact on your training than adding an extra set to your circuit training routine.

Add reps

Rep ranges within sets can have a big impact on the amount of volume that you do in your session. The amount of reps that you do within a set also has a bearing on your fitness result. As a general rule, the more reps you do, the more that exercise will develop stamina and the lower the reps that you are working at, the more that exercise will develop strength.

This rule has one big factor, and that's the resistance level. If you are looking to build strength, you should work at a rep range of 6 – 10 per exercise. For best results with this, resistance level should be at such that you are reaching failure at the end of your planned reps. Failure meaning that you can no longer perform reps in good form.

If you are looking to tone up, burn fat or are looking to develop endurance or stamina in the muscle, aim for 25 – 50 reps at about 50 – 60% of your max resistance level for that exercise.

For general health and function, work between 12 and 15 reps.

Training method

We've covered three different training methods in this guide, but there are many more for you to explore and as many ways to fit them in to your particular lifestyle. As mentioned, you might want to stick to a single training method, as many people do. There is no reason that you can't train in a bunch of different ways. You could even train with all three methods outlined in this book in a single week. This will depend on your goals, however.

If you are considering training sessions that use lots of different methods, think about your goal. If you are serious about achieving a specific result, ask yourself if that training method will benefit you. For example: You wouldn't see a marathon runner training for a marathon by spending their time lifting weights in the gym and you wouldn't see a bodybuilder training for a competition by spending their time outside, running long distance.

Be aware also that it can become easier to lose track and is harder to form exercise habits. I always suggest that along with your exercise plan, you actually book out regular slots per week that you can train in. This way, you are organised; you have a schedule and are prepared. So if you want results, create a structure with your training plan.

Thank you! If you found this useful I'd like to help further...

First off, I would like to thank you for your purchase. It really means a lot that you chose to spend your time on this guide. I am a self-published author with a passion for training and helping people get to where they want to be with fitness and by reading; you are supporting me and fuelling my passion.

This guide should give you a brilliant start into the world of resistance band training and the planning and prep that goes with it. But this is not my first fitness book! I've been writing and self-publishing for several years. I've written books on fitness motivation, planning, bodybuilding, home workouts and long distance running. These guides are based on my experience and formal education.

I've been a long distance, endurance runner, a competing bodybuilder, and I have worked with personal training clients to change their lives through fitness, so I have a lot to share.

If you found this short guide useful and would like to read more about body transformations, fitness motivation, home workouts or more about resistance training and would like a clear path to follow, I have a plenty more for you to look at including workbooks and journals for you to plan and track!

Most of my books are available in eBook and paperback format, and some are also available as audio titles narrated by an awesome voice actor called Matt Addis.

Each fitness book is written as a standalone guide but also has its place as part of a series. So if you are a total beginner and want to become a bodybuilder or marathon runner as an end goal, I have you covered! Jump in at the start of the series with *"Fitness & Exercise Motivation"* and follow the steps. I'll be at the starting blocks with you and we will cross the finish line together!

If you would like to learn more about this series and my other books, you can do so by visiting my author page. Visit Amazon and search "James Atkinson". You will see my ugly mug, click it, and you should be taken to my page.

As we all know, diet plays a big part in health and fitness, and the two subjects fit hand in hand. So I would like to offer you a free download of seven healthy recipes that I created and use regularly myself. You can copy the recipes exactly, add your own twist to them, or simply take inspiration from them.

If you would like to grab this along with other free content such as video tutorials, motivation and fitness planning guides become a part of my email list and we'll reach our fitness goals together! You can do so by following the link below, or using the QR code.

https://yourfitnesssuccess.com/all-the-freebiees/

Don't worry, I never spam, and newsletters are infrequent, but there is always something of value inside when they are sent.

There is a podcast!

Trying to create an online business is tough, especially in the fitness niche! There is a lot of noise, "fairy-tale" fitness supplements, big personalities, and celebrities with huge online followings pushing their fitness ideas that often drown out the information that will actually make the difference.

In an attempt to widen my online reach, I created a podcast that is designed for the beginner who really wants to get results from their efforts. I set out to create bite sized podcast episodes of around twenty minutes that gave honest, actionable advice to the listener. This is still in its early stages, but I have to say that I've absolutely loved doing these podcast episodes and it is something that I plan to get stuck into more in the future.

If you are interested in fitness podcasts, you can find mine at

AudioFitTest.com

Or search Audiofittest wherever you get your podcasts from.

It would be great to have you along! If you do stop by, I would also really appreciate "Likes", "follows" and reviews. These things really help! The same goes for Amazon reviews for the books. If you have a chance and you found the book useful, it would mean the world to me if you left a star rating and a short review.

Thanks again for your support and I wish you all the best with your training. Remember, I am always happy to help where I can, so if you have any questions, just give me a shout!

All the best

Jim

I will leave you with a bit about cardio training ☺…

Cardio training.

Cardio training can range from walking to running, from jogging to circuit training and intervals, so it's a pretty broad subject that wears many faces! Adding some form of cardio is always recommended for everyone. A regular, short, brisk walk can make the world of difference to some.

This book is not about cardio training, but I know for a fact that fitness training can be positively life changing. Cardio is part of fitness and just happens to be the most accessible form of exercise for most people. Walking, jogging, running and sprinting are activities that most of us can get stuck into right away.

Before I was a bodybuilder, I was a long-distance runner and before I was a long-distance runner; I was a cardio failure! The journey from cardio failure to long distance endurance runner was a life changing one for me and I learned a lot from this, so much so that I wrote a bestselling book on the subject.

I want to share a part of this with you now. Here is an excerpt from the book. I hope you enjoy it and find it useful.

CHAPTER 7 - Marathon Training & Distance Running

WHERE TO START

This section is really aimed at the beginner, but it may still hold some useful information for the veteran.

With anything that you do, you have to start from the beginning, and I firmly believe that having a solid foundation to build on is a must if you want results.

It would be great if every goal that you had was achievable overnight, but with any serious fitness goal, the mind-set of progression training is a fundamental factor for success!

Of course, you would not expect to be able to run a marathon in a few short weeks of training. And I would like to clarify that if you are just starting out, there is a long road ahead of you... (Excuse the pun.)

This may sound negative, and many people would be put off by the fact that at least six months of hard, consistent, and smart training will only get them a small step closer to their goal.

I'm talking about the guys that have never done any exercise before and would like to take up the challenge of a marathon.

If you are this guy or gal, I would first like to congratulate you on making this decision and also like to reassure you that you CAN do this.

When you cross that finish line, I'm sure that it will be one of the greatest accomplishments of your life, and your training, character building, and determination leading up to this accomplishment will definitely enrich you as a person.

YOUR FIRST RUN (WHAT TO EXPECT)

The first time you step out of your door, you will probably be motivated, have some shiny new running shoes and training attire, and be ready to start pounding the pavement.

There are a few things that can literally kill your motivation and make you hang up your new running shoes permanently if you are not careful. The biggest killer of your goals in this situation is...

"too much, too soon."

I have seen it, overheard conversations about it, and actually been there myself.

Everything's great. You are all ready to start your marathon training. You have planned your route, you are hydrated, and you know this is going to be the start of something very special! You give a few cursory hamstring stretches and set off on your first run.

Two minutes in and you are fighting for air, your lungs are on fire, you feel sick, and you are wondering how on god's green earth you are even going to finish your first run when you are in this state and you can still see your front door?

Believe me; if you have never felt this way before, you need to actually be there to understand the mental effect that this has on you. It can be devastating!

You will no doubt be able to relate to this feeling very soon as your training progresses. But I will say that it can be controlled, and when you look back at these events, they won't seem that bad. It's just while you are there that you will feel your world is ending!

Before you start your training, please read the Breathing and Running Style chapters. If you can understand and practice this before you even start your first run, it will help you out massively.

YOUR FIRST RUN (WHAT TO DO)

Once you have your breathing and running style sorted, you will be ready for your first run.

The thing is, your first run will not actually be a run! Remember that this is all about progression and you have to start somewhere. If you have never been on a run before, your body isn't used to the kind of stresses put on it, so you will probably end up in the state that we just talked about.

Once you have your route planned out, you should don your trainers and get ready, as you would expect. But your first training session should be a steady walk around your route. This will benefit you more than you probably think.

First of all, it will start you on your routine. Next, it will get you used to your new running shoes. These are a vital piece of kit for any runner.

"Bad shoes = Bad feet, and with bad feet, you can't do a whole lot of running"

Another thing that walking your route will help you with is getting your body used to prolonged activity. These early sessions will also help you to prepare mentally for your training too as you will be able to visualise your route and you will get to know how long this will take you or how close you are to the finish line.

Depending on how fit you are or how quickly you progress, you may want to do this walk for the first full week, but you can assess your progress after your first session.

All that being said, starting off slowly is one thing, but progression is vital if you want to improve and actually reach "long-distance runner status."

This "easy start" approach may be refreshing to some readers, but you also need to progress and push yourself. It may take you a few weeks to find your limits and assess your fitness progression, but this is all part of the process. It is important that you find the right balance.

This is what I would do if I had never done any fitness:

First Session

- Walk my route at a consistent pace

Second Session

- If the previous session was too easy, I would pick up my pace a bit.

- If the previous session was too hard, I would shorten the route a bit.

- If the previous session made me out of breath slightly and had me sweating but I was otherwise comfortable, I would consider a short jogging stint at the last section of my next session.

As you can see, there are a few factors that you can change each time that you train. The important part at this stage is to never sit back and go through the motions; you MUST be progressing. If your sessions do not push you slightly, you will not develop the endurance that you are looking for.

But at this point, there is no need to get to the stage of physical discomfort mentioned at the beginning of this chapter. It will only mess with your mind.

Also by James Atkinson

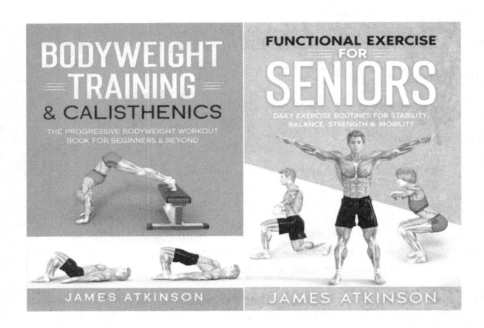

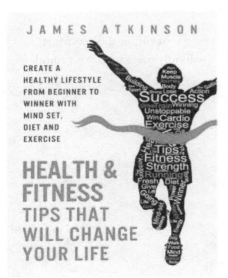

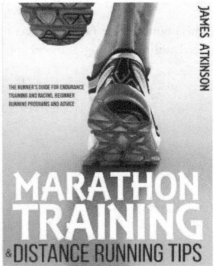

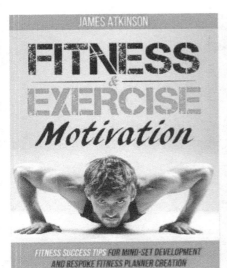

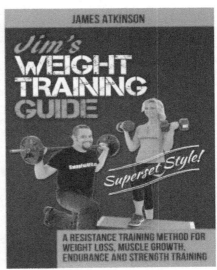

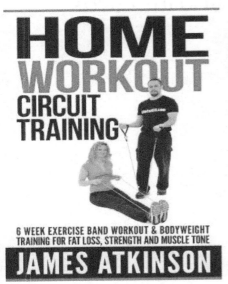

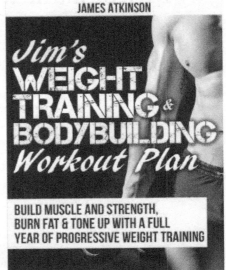

More blank workout cards

MUSCLE GROUP	EXERCISE	RESISTANCE BAND	SETS	REPS

SINGLE EXERCISE

SINGLE EXERCISE				
MUSCLE GROUP	EXERCISE	RESISTANCE BAND	SETS	REPS

SINGLE EXERCISE				
MUSCLE GROUP	EXERCISE	RESISTANCE BAND	SETS	REPS

CIRCUIT TRAINING			
MUSCLE GROUP	EXERCISE	RESISTANCE BAND	REPS

NUMBERS OF CIRCUITS	-	
REST BETWEEN CIRCUITS	-	

CIRCUIT TRAINING			
MUSCLE GROUP	EXERCISE	RESISTANCE BAND	REPS

NUMBERS OF CIRCUITS -	
REST BETWEEN CIRCUITS -	

CIRCUIT TRAINING			
MUSCLE GROUP	EXERCISE	RESISTANCE BAND	REPS

NUMBERS OF CIRCUITS	-	
REST BETWEEN CIRCUITS	-	

SUPERSETS				
SUPERSET	EXERCISES	RESISTANCE BAND	REPS	SETS
#1				
#2				
#3				
#4				
#5				
#6				
#7				

SUPERSET	EXERCISES	RESISTANCE BAND	REPS	SETS
#1				
#2				
#3				
#4				
#5				
#6				
#7				

SUPERSETS				
SUPERSET	EXERCISES	RESISTANCE BAND	REPS	SETS
#1				
#2				
#3				
#4				
#5				
#6				
#7				

Made in the USA
Monee, IL
07 February 2025